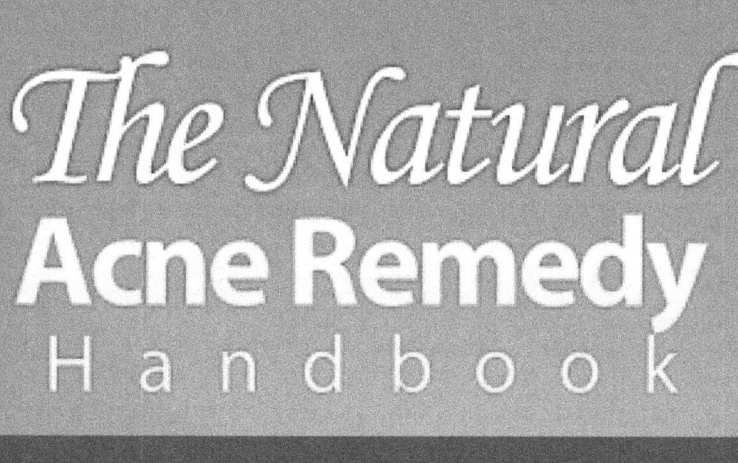

The Natural
Acne Remedy
H a n d b o o k

50 Ways To Treat Acne
Using Natural Remedies

Disclaimer

This e-book has been written for information purposes only. Every effort has been made to make this ebook as complete and accurate as possible. However, there may be mistakes in typography or content. Also, this e-book provides information only up to the publishing date. Therefore, this ebook should be used as a guide - not as the ultimate source.

The purpose of this ebook is to educate. The author and the publisher does not warrant that the information contained in this e-book is fully complete and shall not be responsible for any errors or omissions. The author and publisher shall have neither liability nor responsibility to any person or entity with respect to any loss or damage caused or alleged to be caused directly or indirectly by this e-book.

INTRODUCTION

Acne is a skin disease that involves the oil glands found at the base of hair follicles. These glands come to life during puberty due to both male and female hormones produced at that time. Because of these hormones, this is the time acne usually occurs. Acne occurs when the oil glands at the base of hair follicles get blocked and oil accumulates under the skin.

Acne isn't medically dangerous, but it can be frustrating and embarrassing, especially for teens. It is estimated that nearly ¾ of the population between 11 and 30 will get acne. When acne flares up, it usually occurs on the face, but often can be found on the back, chest, shoulders and neck.

Research shows that susceptibility to get acne may be genetic. If the child's mother had acne, then the child is likely to have it. There are also medications that may cause acne, mainly those that contain androgen and lithium. If you're susceptible to acne, using greasy cosmetics can cause it to flare up. During pregnancy, hormone changes may cause acne to either develop for the first time, or to recur if you had it in the past.

Types of Acne

- Whiteheads—This type of acne remains under the skin and appear very small.

- Blackheads—These are very visible, but you should remember that the blackhead isn't caused by dirt, and no matter how well you clean your face, the blackheads won't go away.

- Papules—Small pink bumps visible on the surface of the skin.

- Pustules—Red bumps visible on the skin that have pus at the top.

- Nobules—Large solid pimples that are painful. They are formed deep in the skin.

- Cysts—They can easily scar the skin surface. Cysts are painful and pus filled.

You go to the movies and see beautiful people on the screen with glowing perfect skin. Perhaps you've even envied those people. In reality, however, their skin might not be as "perfect" as you think. Many famous people such as Jessica Simpson, Kelly Clarkson, and Katy Perry have all confessed to being plagued with acne. Sure, stage makeup gives them that "glowing" skin, but underneath they had the same skin care problem many people around the world face—dreaded acne.

As previously stated, when puberty hits, so do the zits. Hormones rage and many hormones can actually cause acne to occur. At that age, even one pimple can seem devastating. For some, their acne problems are just a small amount of acne that goes away rather quickly. For others, however, it can be a nightmare. Acne seems to take over their face, and nothing they buy seems to work. Some are even troubled with it through adulthood. Often, these individuals have it so badly that they are scarred for the rest of their lives. Acne can not only be a burden, it can be extremely embarrassing for those who have it. This is especially so during your teen years when self-esteem is so important. Face it, sometimes kids can be cruel, and those with severe cases of acne can be a target. They get harassed and/or made fun of. This really stresses them out, which makes the acne even worse. It can be a vicious cycle.

When you're one of those people tormented with acne, what can you do? You see so many commercials telling you to buy this product or use this cleanser and rid yourself of acne. It can be confusing trying to figure out what to buy. Some people spend hundreds of dollars trying to find the right product. They end up buying a lot of products that never seem to work.

Treatment for acne can include over-the-counter creams or gels which usually include benzoyl peroxide to remove dead skin cells and prevent clogging or salicylic acid to unclog pores.

Prescription medications can include oral antibiotics or topical antimicrobials that help reduce acne-causing bacteria. For women, prescription medication can include contraceptives that calm sebum producing glands and reduce oil.

If these don't work, then physical procedures can be performed by your doctor. These usually include chemical peels that unclog pores and remove dead skin cells.

If you go this route, be careful when choosing a dermatologist. Not all of them are experienced with acne. Check them out and ask them to show you photographs of patients who have used the treatment they recommend for you. They should be able to show you before and after shots.

If you've never had acne problems, you probably have no idea how expensive medical treatment can be. Here are just a few of the costs you can incur if you go the medicinal route to acne skin care:

- Over-the-counter regimens that include a cleanser, a toner and a medicated lotion that is not prescribed and used daily can cost from $30-$60 per month.

- If it's severe and your doctor prescribes antibiotics, topical creams, ointments or hormone therapy the treatment can cost anywhere from $50-$200 per month with a doctor visit.

- Others try acne treatments that include facials or chemical peels. These treatments can cost anywhere from $75 to $200 for each session, and may require more than one session in a month.

- Some people who suffer from acne become scarred by it. Often, these patients choose to endure additional treatments to remove or lessen the appearance of acne scars. Both microdermabrasion and dermabrasion are used for the scaring and can cost up to $2,000 when more than one treatment is needed.

After the acne clears up using the medical treatments, you have to continue the medical treatment so it won't flare up again. Sometimes, these medical treatments are considered cosmetic and are not covered by insurance. Doctors will sometimes provide discounts for skin resurfacing treatments for their new patients. They may also offer package deals if you need multiple treatments. You can also often find prescription drugs that are generic. These can cost you up to 50% less.

Here are a few specific medical treatment options and their costs:

- Tretinoin—Depending on the strength, it can cost you anywhere between $35 and $50 dollars for a 45 gram tube.

- Adapalene—this is generic and comes in different strengths. It is quite expensive. It can cost you approximately $160 for a 45 gram tube.

- Epiduo—This combines adapalene with benzoyl peroxide. For a 45 gram tube of this gel, it can cost up to $250. You can buy benzoyl peroxide cheaply, so it may not be worth it to you to pay this much for the combination of the antibiotic and the benzoyl peroxide.

- Retin-A Micro—This may cause less irritation and is a microsphere preparation of trentinoin. A 45 Gram tube can cost between $260 and $320. Avita is also a form of trentinon and is a bit cheaper ranging from $150-$175 for 45 grams.

- Tazorac treats acne and psoriasis. It is considered effective, but is also irritating. For only 30 grams of this gel, you can expect to pay between $200 and $250.

- Benzaclin—1% clindamycin and 5% benzoyl peroxide—This is a little more affordable. It costs between $75 and $90 for a tube that is 25 grams.

- Duac—A brand-name gel that is virtually the same as Benzaclin, but is more expensive. For 45 grams, it can cost you over $200.

- Ziana—It is expensive, between $225 and $250 for only 30 grams. If you mix two generics—clindamycin and tretinoin—you can expect to pay somewhere between $50 and $100 for both of them.

- Doxycycline—This is a prescription pill where you take 50 mg to 100 mg two times a day. It's generic and you can usually get it for $4 for the entire month's supply.

- Oracea—This is a 40 mg tablet to treat acne. It is effective, but is expensive. It can cost you $400 for a month's supply.

- Minocycline—This medication is taken twice a day and is less likely to give you a rash with exposure to sun than doxycycline. For 50 mg to 100 mg doses, you can buy it for as low as $12 to $30 for a full month's supply.

- Solodyn—This is minocycline in an extended release form. While it is more convenient than daily dosing, it can cost you anywhere from $560 to $1,000 depending on the dose.

As you can see, acne sufferers can spend a lot of money. Often, it's wasted because the creams and pills don't work. You may have tried many of them yourself and feel like you're spending all your money trying to clear your skin to no avail.

What if there was a way you could rid yourself of acne and you wouldn't have to spend a penny, would you try it? You may find this to be the case. In fact, you just might have something in the kitchen or bathroom cabinets that will work just fine.

It's frustrating when you feel you don't have control of what is happening to your face. People try everything over-the-counter and take every medication their dermatologist gives them and still have terrible acne breakouts. Sometimes, however, the answer isn't in dermatologists or medications. Instead, the answer is found in nature. Natural remedies have been found to help clear up acne. They're less harmful to your skin, and can be just as effective, or even more effective, as the products you spend a lot of money on.

50 WAYS TO TREAT ACNE USING NATURAL REMEDIES

If you're one of those who suffer from severe acne, you're probably willing to try just about anything. If you've tried and tried to clear your face of acne and you've used every cleanser or acne cream you can think of and you are still plagued with acne, you should know that there are many natural ways to help you clear up your acne and often get rid of it permanently. You don't have to waste money, and most of these things you already have around your house. If you think this sounds too good to be true, trust me, it isn't.

You can have clearer skin in a short period of time for far less money than you'd spend buying medical creams and pills. Often, you don't have to use anything. You just have to adjust a few things that you do in your daily routine to help clear up your acne. Wouldn't that be awesome? Natural remedies have worked for others, and these remedies can work for you too. Try several of these methods until you find the combination of natural products that work for you.

Here are 50 tips you can use that will naturally help you clear up that dreaded acne and reclaim healthy, clear skin:

1.	Baking Soda—When you think baking soda, you probably think of keeping your refrigerator fresh. Baking soda, in fact, does much more. For acne, mix baking soda and water in equal parts. Use them to make a paste you can apply to your face. Don't put it all over your face. You'll only want to put it on each individual acne spot. It's usually easier to use a Q-Tip and dab it on. Leave it on your face until it dries. This usually takes around 10 minutes. Wash it off in water that is very cold. This helps close pores. Generally, doing this twice each day can give results.

2. Lemon Juice—Lemons have citric acid which fights bacteria that cause acne. It's easy to use as an acne treatment. Simply cut a lemon in half. Then rub the open side of the lemon gently on your face. You will feel it stinging, which mean it is working. Leave it on for about 10 minutes. Be sure to wash the lemon juice off. When you use lemon juice for your acne, you probably should use sunscreen if you're going outdoors. The citric acid can sometimes bleach the skin. This can make your skin more sensitive and makes it a higher risk for sun damage.

3. Potatoes—Slice a small, raw potato in half. Rub it on the acne. You want to rub it only on the affected areas, not your entire face. Potatoes not only have a healing effect, but are also an anti-inflammatory. This will help with that embarrassing and irritating swelling and redness acne can have on your face.

When you're finished, wash the potato residue off of your face gently.

4. Toothpaste—This works well for pimples. If you have one or two that you want to get rid of quickly, simply apply toothpaste to it. Toothpaste contains silica which dries out and reduces the size of the pimple overnight if you leave it on. Toothpaste that has silica but not sodium lauryl sulfate works best. Most big name-brand toothpastes have sodium lauryl sulfate, so stick with the simple, natural ones when you use it to treat your acne.

5. Ice—Ice has been used for years to treat inflammation in the body. That's why when there's swelling from any kind of an injury, ice is applied to the affected area. For acne, ice is used because it closes pores as well as helps reduce the inflammation of acne. If you have big pores, you can take ice cubes and rub them gently over the problem spots. Ice or even cold packs, work to constrict blood vessels beneath the skin. This causes irritation and/or inflammation to be less noticeable.

6. Tea Tree Oil—It is a well-known anti-fungal and antibacterial remedy. It's herbal, so it's great for mild-moderate acne. In tests, it has been just as effective as benzoyl peroxide for acne. The benzoyl peroxide may work more quickly, but teal tree oil

12

will have fewer side effects and treat your acne naturally.

7.	Aspirin—You'll want to crush the aspirin and form a paste. Then use a Q-Tip or your finger to apply the paste on each pimple and let it dry. Aspirin contains salicylic acid. They use this in most acne treatments, because it will destroy bacteria which cause acne. It dries out pimples while it fights bacteria. Leave the mixture on your face for 10-15 minutes and wash off gently.

8.	Alum—You can check the spice aisle in your local grocery store and look for Potassium alum. It is also used in natural deodorants and styptic to help reduce bleeding after a cut because it's a natural antiseptic and astringent that shrinks skin tissue. It works better in block form than power. Just wipe it over your acne gently to avoid irritating pimples.

9.	Reduce refined carbohydrates from your diet—Things like bread, pasta, etc. can cause your acne to worsen. You should also try to cut back on sugar. You may want to use a little natural sugar, but eating a lot of sweets will negatively affect your acne. When you're looking for something to munch on, instead of candy bars, go for things that are healthier, such as fruits and vegetables.

10.	Fermented foods—Foods such as sauerkraut, kefir, natural yogurt or goat cheese contain pro-biotic and enzymes which help reduce acne. Adding these to your diet can be beneficial when you're struggling with acne breakouts.

11. Stop using products on your face such as cleansers, makeup, and face cream—If you feel you need these things, you should look until you find natural products. Often these products aren't made to work together. If you're trying natural ways to cure your acne, then don't counteract the effect with other chemical products.

12. Vegetables—You've been told all your life it's important to eat your vegetables. If you have acne problems, you should definitely add more vegetables to your daily diet. They're healthy, and they clean toxins from your blood that can cause acne.

13. Water—Drinking water also helps cleanse the body. You should try to get about half your body weight in ounces of water daily. As the water cleanses your body, it will help cleanse the pores of the skin and keep them from clogging. If you drink more water instead of soft drinks, you'll probably not only see a difference in your acne, but your health in general.

14. Be active—Moving around helps your lymphatic system. Try doing things such as running, jumping rope, or even jumping on a trampoline. Join a gym and workout. Join a sports team in school or at your local YMCA. Whatever activity you enjoy that gets you moving. Often when one suffers from acne they stay home and seem to become a young couch potato. They don't want to go anywhere or do anything where others will see their acne. Forget about that. Don't worry about others, worry about yourself. You need to move, so get out and do it. Run laps around your yard if necessary, but move!

15. Vitamin A—Taking a multivitamin is good whether or not you have acne, but it is proven that Vitamin A does help reduce acne. You should try to get a vitamin that has a good supply of Vitamin A, because it helps regenerate skin. It can reduce wrinkles and help get rid of blemishes.

16. Keep your face clean—You can use simple soap and wash your face at least twice a day. If your skin tends to be oily, you should rinse it several times throughout the day. Use lukewarm water to help remove oil that leads to breakouts. You should use mild soap and a soft washcloth or soft sponge. Strong soaps and rough material will irritate acne. Just a little soap is enough. Make sure you rinse it thoroughly. After washing splash your face with cool water to close your pores. When

you're finished, pat your face dry—don't rub it.

17. Sleep well—The more you sleep, the less stressed you'll be. Every hour you lose of sleep causes you around 15% more stress. This can cause the hormones to go crazy causing acne. Instead of staying up late watching TV, or cramming for that test you forgot to study for, you should go to bed at a decent hour.

18. No popping or picking—If you're doing everything you can using natural remedies to treat your acne, it can be useless if you pop or pick at your acne. You may want to, but it won't be good for you in the long run. Acne is bacteria and when you pop it, you allow it to spread to more pores. In effect, you're spreading bacteria to the pores you just cleaned. That's not a good idea. Popping and picking acne also causes inflammation which can cause the acne to appear worse, and cause you to have scars.

19. Avoid glycemic foods—Foods with high glycemic content are not good for acne. This includes: soft drinks, white bread, rice, potatoes, beer, cake, and commercial cereals to name a few. Making a few changes in your diet, like substituting a baked sweet potato for your usual loaded baked potato, eating whole wheat cereals, or buying pasta enriched with soy protein can help reduce your glycemic intake.

20. Baby powder—Baby powder has long been used to absorb moisture. Lightly rub your face with baby powder before you go to bed and when you get up in the morning. The baby powder will keep your face dry and oil-free and will help dry up blemishes.

21. Honey—Use a honey mask on your face a few times a week. Honey is an antibacterial, and can disinfect and help heal blemishes. It is gentle enough for even the most sensitive skin. You use the honey like you would any commercial facial mask. Just rub the honey on your entire face. Let it sit until it's totally dry, and then peel it off.

22. Keep your hair away—Your hair contains oil and can help lead to breakouts. Wash your hair everyday and after every workout. If your hair is long or you have bangs, be sure to pull your hair away from your face. Cleaning your face and then allowing your hair to be on it can reduce the effect of your cleansing. Many people use their hair to hide their acne. They keep their hair over as much of their face as possible. You're not the first person to have severe acne, and you won't be the last. Pull your hair back and don't worry who sees it. You may be self conscious at first, but when your acne begins to clear, you'll be glad you did it.

23. Eat carrots—Carrots have beta-carotene or Vitamin A—They help strengthen your protective tissue and prevent acne. It is also a good antioxidant which can help rid your body of toxins. Carrots are great for a snack and are much better to nibble on while you do your homework than chips or cookies.

24. Clean pillowcases—Your face lays on your pillow daily. The pillowcase can absorb oil from your skin. If your wash your face before you go to bed and lay your head on a dirty pillowcase, you're reapplying the dirt and oil. This renders your cleansing useless. You should wash your pillowcase at least every other day. This way, you will get the most from your natural treatments.

25. Eat foods with Zinc—Look for foods that are high in Zinc. It is an antibacterial agent necessary in your skin's oil-producing. Not getting enough Zinc can actually cause breakouts. There are many foods high in Zinc such as: oysters, wheat germ, veal liver, roast beef, roasted pumpkin and squash, dark chocolate, lamb, peanuts, and crab. Adding some of these to your diet can help fight your acne.

26. Avoid smoking—You know smoking is bad for you. It damages many parts of your body and causes multiple health problems.

For acne, smoking can clog pores and increase breakouts.

27. No excessive sunbathing—Some sun is good for you, but if you're going to be in the sun for some time, be sure to wear SPF. You're probably using a lot of products either commercial or natural on your face. Many of these react to extreme sunlight. Using SPF will help take care of your skin.

28. Rose water glycerine—Rose water glycerine makes a good facial rinse. After cleaning your face, using rose water glycerine as a rinse can help remove residue and other pollutants. It leaves your face cleaner than just with soap and water.

29. Don't touch—You have no idea how many surfaces your hands touch each day. They are constantly in contact with dirt and germs. When you touch your face, rub your eyes, etc, you just transfer all of that dirt and germs onto your face. It's a good idea to wash your hands frequently as a general rule of health. If you find it difficult not to touch your face, make sure you wash your hands often. If possible, however, avoid touching your face.

30. Don't drink alcohol—Excessive consumption of alcohol can enlarge the blood vessels that are near your skins surface.

31. Don't use multiple skincare products—You should never mix any kind of products from your pharmacy, including skincare products. Some don't work well with others. Others will have the same ingredients. This means you're getting too much of it and can help increase the problem. If you find a skincare product that works, stick with it and get rid of the others. Once you find natural ways to cleanse your face and prevent acne that work, just do away with the store-bought ones.

32. Grapeseed oil—Add a teaspoon of grapeseed oil to whichever toner you use. It can help your skin cells damaged by acne repair themselves.

33. Apple cider vinegar/rubbing alcohol/lemon juice toner—Don't mix them together, but individually, these work well. These both kill dead skin cells and clean out pores because they are highly acidic. You do have to be careful when you use them. If your skin starts to dry out, you can use the one you choose less often or use water to dilute it a bit.

34. Brown sugar—When you take a shower and your skin is damp it causes your pores to open up. Use brown sugar and scrub the acne areas. It helps with acne and helps keep your skin smooth. You don't want to use the scrub every day. Two or three times a

month is sufficient.

35. Egg whites—They help remove oil from your skin. You just crack one or two eggs and separate the whites. Beat the whites until they are consistent. Spread the whites over your face and keep it on for 15-20 minutes and then wash off. It will help leave your skin oil-free, which will definitely help fight acne.

36. Egg yolks—The yolks help stop pores from becoming clogged. They have Vitamin A comprised of retinoids. You find this Retin-A in many beauty products. Mix up the yolks and put them on your face. Let them harden and then keep on your face for 15-20 minutes, and then wash off. Doing this at least once a week will help prevent pore clogging.

37. Garlic—While this hasn't been proven scientifically, it has been known to work. Simply peel two garlic cloves and smash them into a pulp. Use the juice squeezed out of it to apply to your face. Leave it on for five to 10 minutes. You can use it as often as you want, but don't leave it on too long at a time.

38. Mint—Mint can soothe your skin. They contain menthol, which is an anti-inflammatory. They help take away that red your skin shows when you have acne. Either use the juice of mint tea

leaves or mint oil. Put it on your face for 10-15 minutes and rinse off. You can use it as many times as you want, and since it's an anti-inflammatory, it won't hurt your skin.

39. Cinnamon and honey mixture—Take one teaspoon of each and mix it together. Put it on your face and let it sit for 15 minutes. Rinse with warm water and pat dry. Cinnamon has many good properties such as antiviral, antifungal, and antibacterial. Honey is a natural antiseptic, so it can heal and soothe. It's a hygroscopic as well, so it can absorb moisture.

40. Plain yogurt—If you know how, it's better to make your own yogurt than to buy it from the shelves. You want to use plain yogurt either way. Make a yogurt face pack and leave it on your skin for about 20 minutes. Wash it off with warm water. It helps cleanse your skin and is cooling and soothing.

41. Acne facial oil that is homemade—Mixing natural oils can give you a good facial oil to help moisturize your skin. You can use about one ounce of jojoba oil. Add 3 drops each of carrot seed oil, lavender oil, and geranium oil. Mix them all together and rub a small amount of the mixture between your fingertips and lightly apply the oil to your face.

42. Clove oil—You don't want to put straight clove oil on your face, because it will burn. Find a good clove oil blend. It helps with the severe cystic acne. It's a topical treatment that can help reduce acne overnight.

43. Loosen athletic wear—Wearing headbands or helmets, for example, can cause excessive acne around the hairline. Helmets can also cause them on the skin near the chin strap because it rubs the skin. If you must wear either of these for athletic reasons, try loosening them a bit or taking them off when they're not in use to let the skin breathe.

44. Shower after any kind of workout—Whether you go to a gym, play football, shoot hoops with your friends, play tennis, or jog, your body sweats. When it does, it helps remove dead skin cells. That's good, and the activity is definitely needed to help with acne, but the sweat leaves salt behind on your body. You need to wash it off or the salt will clog those recently cleaned pores.

45. Learn to manage your stress—Stress, especially during your teen years, can be heavy. Sometimes you stress out over acne. This only increases your breakouts. When you're stressed, your body releases stress hormones. It causes you to increase oil levels in your body and greatly affects the skin. Find some

activity that helps relax you and reduces your stress. Taking walks and using them to clear your head often helps. Preparing for tests in advance instead of last minute cramming helps as well as making sure your assignments aren't rush jobs does. Anything that can cause you to have pressure on you and causes you to stress out needs to be dealt with and managed properly.

46. Turmeric—You'll find this spice in Indian food. When you're cooking at home, you can spice up your food if you can add it to things like eggs or stir-fry. It has anti-inflammatory, antiseptic, and antimicrobial properties. It can reduce the inflammation and redness of your acne.

47. Keep things that touch your face clean—Be sure your cell phone, sunglasses or regular glasses or anything else that touches your face is cleaned with anti-bacterial wipes that are safe for devices. Just as you don't want to touch your face with dirty hands, you don't want to touch it with dirty devices. You don't want to do anything to reclog the pores you've just cleaned.

48. Reduce dairy intake—Studies have shown that if you have too much dairy you can cause oil glands to produce more oil which is bad for your acne. You can substitute some products such as

soy or coconut milk for regular milk to help reduce the intake and keep your oil at a minimum.

49. Banana peels—Try taking a small piece of banana peel and rubbing it on the acne for a few minutes. Rub it until the inside of the peel turns brown. As the peel particles dry on you or face, your skin absorbs the nutrients and vitamins in the peel. Leave it on for about 30 minutes and wash it off in warm water. Do this three times a day. At night, when you use it, it's alright to leave the peel particles on your face overnight and wash it off the next morning.

50. Papaya—They use Papaya in many beauty products you see advertised today.   You don't, however, have to buy a lot of products to get the benefit of Papaya.   Raw papaya works even better, and it's a natural acne remedy. It will help remove dead skin cells as well as excess lipids from the skin. Papa also helps with inflammation, due to the enzyme papain which it contains. It's easy to use. Simply rinse your face with water and pat it dry. Take the flesh of a papaya and mash it thoroughly. You'll want it to have a consistency that you can apply to your skin. Put it on the affected areas. Allow it to remain on your skin for approximately 20 minutes and then rinse it off. Use warm water and pat dry. If your skin dries out after you cleanse, you should find a natural moisturizer that is appropriate for the type of skin.

you have and use it afterward. This will help take care of your skin.

If you're wondering about the costs of natural treatments, you may be surprised in the difference between medicinal and natural treatments. Here are a few examples of the costs of natural acne fighting treatments:

- A box of Arm & Hammer baking soda costs under $2.00 just about anywhere you shop, and since you only use a small amount, it can go a long way.

- Lemons—Depending on where you live and what season it is, lemons can be purchased from $.50 to $1.00 each. If you acne is mild, you don't even have to use ½ a lemon. You can slice one in several pieces.

- Toothpaste—You can check inexpensive toothpastes to see if they have sodium lauryl sulfate. If they do, you can buy a tube of all natural toothpaste for around $5. You only use a very small amount, so a tube goes a long way.

- Potatoes—Almost every home has potatoes, so it isn't an added expense to use one on your face. You can buy potatoes almost anywhere for an average of $.50 a pound.

- Honey—The average bottle of honey costs around $6. If you want to use the cinnamon and honey mix, you can actually buy cinnamon honey for the same price.

- Cinnamon—A name-brand bottle of cinnamon can sometimes costs around $5. You can find generic versions at most grocery or discount stores for much less.

- Aspirin—You can get a large bottle of over 100 tablets at your local Dollar Tree. Paying $1 is a small price to pay to give it a try.

- Baby powder—It doesn't matter if it's name-brand or generic. Generic versions can be found at Dollar Tree.

- Grapeseed oil—A 16 oz bottle can be purchased for around $10. You only use a small amount, so it will go a long way.

- Brown Sugar—A two-pound box of Domino brown sugar costs around $1.20. Off-brand costs even less.

- Eggs—On the average, eggs costs about $1.50 per dozen. Since you don't use them daily, and can use both the whites and the yolks to treat your acne, that's a full-month's supply.

- Garlic—The average costs of garlic cloves is around $1.80 per pound.

- Mint—You can buy a 6 oz bottle of mint leaves for under $2.50.

- Rose Water Glycerin—For under $6, you can buy an 8 oz bottle.

- Clove Oil—This is potent and goes a long way. Depending on where you get it and what size you get, you can get a bottle of clove oil for as little as $2. Clove oil that is sold for a beauty product, however, can cost as much as $15.

- Apple Cider Vinegar—At your local Walmart, you can get their brand at the low cost of around $4 for a whole gallon.

- Rubbing Alcohol—You can find a 16-oz bottle for under $4 just about anywhere you look. Sometimes, they have products like this at Dollar Tree, so always check their first.

- Lemon Juice—In an online grocery store, you can buy ReaLemon 100% lemon juice for only $3.39 cents for a 48 oz. bottle.

- Turmeric—McCormick brand ground turmeric comes in 2 oz bottles for around $5.

- Alum—McCormick brand comes in 1.9 oz bottles and costs around $3.

- Vitamin A—While it's good to get this vitamin through the foods you eat, you can buy the supplement in bottles of 250 soft gels for under $4.

- Carrots—Baby carrots are great for snacking, and you can buy a 16 oz bag at ShopRite for only $1.50.

- Bananas—Bananas are a healthy snack. You can buy them for as little as $.30-$.40 cents per pound and then use the peels to help improve your acne. That's a win/win!

- Papayas—These are a little more expensive as far as fruits go. Depending on where you live and the season, you can usually purchase a papaya for around $3. It may cost a little more than other natural treatments, but can be well worth the cost in effectiveness.

If you add the entire cost of each of the above items, you get a little over $65. Wow! That is cheaper than purchasing one of many of the medicinal products. That's so inexpensive you can surely try every one of them to see which ones work for you. Some of them may not work for your type of acne, but others will. With all your choices, the chances of you not being able to find one that works for you is very slim. If you add these natural products to the things you can do and not do in your everyday live to improve your acne naturally, you will surely find a winning combination somewhere.

As you can see, there are numerous natural ways to fight acne. You may be wondering why you should use the natural things instead of just buying a tube of this or a jar of that. There are benefits to using natural methods to treat acne breakouts. Here are a few of them:

- Save Money—As I've clearly shown in the above text, natural remedies are much cheaper than medicine or medical treatments that are available. With the economy today, everyone wants to save money, and medicinal methods of acne control can burn through your wallet quickly. By saving money, you have more to spend on the other things you want.

- Saves Time—When acne gets really bad, most people look for a doctor. If you've ever tried it, it can be exhausting. It can also be heartbreaking when you go to one and then another and they don't help. Finding the right doctor is a process of trial and error that can be costly and take a lot of valuable time. If, however, you use natural treatments, it's as simple as picking up a few extra things while you're at the grocery store. No time is added, and you can spend your time doing things you enjoy instead of waiting in doctor waiting rooms or at the pharmacy for a prescription.

- No Side Effects—Most medications, even if they do work for acne, are toxic pharmaceuticals. They can cause side effects that are actually worse than the acne you're using them to treat. Trying natural methods should always be done before any pharmaceutical method is used. If you use natural, herbal methods to fight your acne, you won't be harming your body. You can rest assured that your body will remain toxic-free. Natural acne treatments are both safe and reliable.

- Boosts Your Self-Esteem—Acne can make your self-esteem crash. You can go from being outgoing and popular to a wall flower who doesn't want to be seen. If you find a natural treatment that helps clear up your acne, your self-esteem will definitely improve.

- Stress Reducer—You may think it sounds silly, but it is actually true that sometimes you stress so much over acne that you won't believe how relieved you'll be when you find a natural remedy that actually works for you. It's like taking a huge weight off of your shoulders and you feel happy and free to get on with your life as a brand new person.

Natural Methods Also Treat Acne Scarring

If you've had acne for a long time, it is likely that you'll have some scaring from it. Scars can be almost as embarrassing as the acne, and can continue your low self-esteem issues. Believe it or not, natural remedies aren't just good for the acne. There are several things you can use for acne that you can also use to get rid of those ugly scars the acne left behind.

- Mint—If you take a bunch of mint leaves and clean them thoroughly. Place them in a soft clean cotton cloth. Twist them until the juice comes out. Take the juice and apply it on the scarred areas and leave it on until it dries thoroughly. After it is dry, simply wash it off and pat it dry. Do this once a day for a month. At the end of the month, you'll begin to see a difference in the appearance of your scars.

- Vitamin E and Aloe Vera—Vitamin E has long been known to help skin. When you put it on the scarred area, it absorbs quickly into your skin and begins to slowly fight the scarring. If you combine the Vitamin E with Aloe Vera, you can fight scars that are both shallow and deep at the same time.

- Lemon—The citric acid in lemons can be used to lighten the skin. When you do this, it naturally lightens the scars. It's the same basic principle you use when using lemons to help cure acne. Just cut the lemon and rub the juice on your scarred areas. Leave it on until it dries thoroughly. Wash it off and pat dry. Don't use this process every day, because it may cause your skin to dry. You can, however, use it about three times a week. Before long, you'll begin to see results.

- Tea tree oil—Like lemons, tea tree oil can be used to cure acne and to reduce scarring. It is found in just about any grocery store. When you put tea tree oil on your skin, it sooths the skin. If you use it daily on your scarred areas, you'll see the scars begin to fade away.

- Tomatoes—They are used to treat acne scars, because tomatoes are the skin correctors. They remove the pigmentation and improve your skin tone. Take a small tomato and cut it in half. Rub the tomato over the damaged, scarred area thoroughly. Leave it on for about 30 minutes. Wash it off completely and pat your face dry.

Nature provides us with everything we need to remain healthy if we know where to look and what to look for. You were born to have clear, acne-free skin. You just need to find Nature's way of giving it to you. It may take a little bit of inexpensive trial and error, but in the long run, it will be worth it. Give it a try. After all, what have you got to lose?

www.ingramcontent.com/pod-product-compliance
Lightning Source LLC
Chambersburg PA
CBHW080354290526
45791CB00009BA/2868